Simple Ways to Have a Balanced Mental Health

How to Improve Mental Health

[RS Johnson]

Table of Contents

Introduction 4

Mental Health in Workplace 6

Our work..8

Our lifestyle... 19

    Exercise... 19

    Relaxation 19

    Creative Ideas for Maintaining and Improving Well-Being keep physically fit 20

Our social relationships 29

    Ways to stay connected................................ 29

Our thoughts.. 34

    Learning the connection between thoughts and feelings 34

Symptoms of common mental health conditions 37

    Anxiety.. 37

    Depression 37

Conclusion.. 38

Introduction

A positive concept known as mental health is defined as the well-being of a person or a community. The concept is concerned with the enjoyment of life, the ability to cope with stress and sadness, the achievement of goals and potential, and a sense of connection to others. Mental health is more about wellness than illness, and it is more than just the absence of a mental health condition. Just as with mental health, physical health is not fixed. Mental health exists from positive, spectrum, healthy functioning to severe symptoms of mental health conditions on others. Throughout a person's life, their mental health fluctuates along this spectrum in response to various stressors and circumstances. People at the green end of the spectrum are healthy, with high levels of resilience and well-being. People may have difficulty coping as they move into the yellow zone. People in the orange zone have more difficulty coping, and symptoms may become more severe and frequent. People at the red end of the spectrum are likely to be experiencing severe symptoms and may be contemplating self-harm or suicide. Risk factors and protective factors have an impact on mental health and can shift people along the continuum. They can be personal or related to family, work, or other aspects of one's life. Risk factors can put additional strain on our mental health, whereas protective factors can help us stay or get better. With so much of people's time spent at work each day, the workplace is a powerful environment for mental health and well-being. A positive and supportive work environment can mean the difference between being 'in the green' and being 'in the orange.'

Mental Health in Workplace

Work can be beneficial to our mental health. It can boost our self-esteem and provide us with a sense of purpose. It properly allows us to interact with others and access resources that we might not have outside of work. On the other hand, factors such as job stress, bullying, and discrimination can hurt our mental health, potentially triggering a mental health condition or worsening an existing condition. When we talk about mental health in the workplace, we mean how our working environment affects us – whether positively or negatively –our ability to do our jobs and our overall well-being.

So, in other words, we should investigate how we do our jobs while also understanding that it is equally important to maintain mental health outside of the workplace. Stress is a normal part of life, and it isn't always a bad thing. A little stress, such as the stress we experience during a job interview, can sometimes help us perform better. However, it is usually only temporary and can assist us in focusing and performing well under pressure. Even if you work under heavy workloads, tight deadlines, or suffer from workplace culture, workplace stress will still make you feel stressed at work.

When workplace stress becomes intense, comes from multiple sources, or lasts for an extended period, it can increase physical and mental health risks or worsen an existing condition.

There is often work-related stress that must be managed, but we must also remember to monitor the stresses in our personal lives. Learning to recognize when we are stressed to avoid or manage the situation is important for staying healthy. Everyone is unique, with different roles at home and work. There is no one best way to stay mentally healthy, but there are several things we can do every day to improve our well-being. Keeping our mental health in good shape necessitates an examination of four key areas of our lives, which are covered in the following chapters:

- Our thoughts
- Our lifestyle
- Our work
- Our social relationships

Our work

At work, many factors outside of our control determine our level of mental well-being, but everyone can properly take steps to improve their mental health and well-being. To assist in their work roles, all employees, including managers, can use some common strategies.

1. Limit working extra hours

Intense periods of activity at work can properly prevent us from working standard hours. However, long hours can hurt our health when they become the norm rather than the exception. Try to keep your overtime to a minimum. Discuss your responsibilities with your manager if working extra hours is becoming more common.

2. Schedule meetings in core work hours

Scheduling meetings to begin and end only during core working hours allows you to work with the confidence that your "out-of-hours" times will be protected, allowing you to plan accordingly. In addition, common email diary systems enable you to block out times in your calendar so that meeting organizers who have access to your calendar are aware of your commitments.

3. Take regular breaks

Getting some fresh air and properly leaving your workplace, or simply moving away from your work area, can help you be more productive.

Some suggestions for vacations

Take an hourly break to increase work productivity. Taking frequent breaks allows the mind and body to recharge. Working breaks also have the following advantages:

- Accidents and injuries in the workplace occur as a result of inattention. As a result, employee productivity increases significantly, increasing company profits.
- Posture can improve as a result of prolonged work at a desk or machine.
- Employee morale rises.

It is very important to take breaks throughout the day properly. However, taking a short break even if machines and computers are idle will still improve productivity. The brief break allows employees to stretch tired muscles, find relief from prolonged positions and postures, and retain any information they may have learned in the previous hour or so.

Short breaks also allow employees to refresh, which reduces costly workplace accidents. Therefore, employees' time during the working day is as important as how frequently and long they take their breaks.

Leave the office during lunch to recharge your batteries for the afternoon.

• Exercise at lunchtime to increase productivity for the rest of the afternoon • Take breaks to help you refocus • Take an afternoon tea break that provides more than just caffeine

Workers frequently rush to the vending machines and coffee pot as soon as break time arrives. To help ensure they have enough energy to get through the rest of the day, they prefer to consume sugar and caffeine before the end of their break. Thus, to prevent fatigue before the next scheduled break, this approach is completely ineffective. And what is more, if this behavior is repeatedly exhibited, it will result in an increase in energy followed by a huge crash, with numerous negative repercussions. But when spent in this manner, breaks do not increase productivity.

Encourage employees to spend their free time on the job in different ways when you want to maximize breaks' effectiveness. The break room environment should be designed to provide employees with the opportunity to relax and rejuvenate.

Consider the following suggestions:

- Make a meditation space. Providing a quiet area for employees to spend a few minutes relaxing and clearing their minds, if there is space, will have a significant impact on productivity.
- In vending machines, swap out junk food for healthy snacks. Some corporations have formed partnerships with local businesses to keep breakrooms and vending machines stocked with nutritious snacks.

Healthy foods provide energy without the fatigue and irritability that sugar and caffeine can cause.

- Schedule exercise breaks in the afternoon.
- Workplace fatigue typically sets in in the afternoon or halfway to two-thirds of the way through a shift. Exercise breaks provide a slew of advantages for your team, one of which is increased productivity. (Learn why Forbes compensates their employees for taking exercise breaks.) It can range from stretching exercises to jumping jacks to allowing employees to mingle and laugh together.

Take Advantage of Microbreaks

Taking 15-minute breaks throughout the day is not always possible. When this occurs, take advantage of microbreaks, which can range from several minutes to several seconds. Microbreaks are still an effective way to mentally or physically relax and reset before returning to your tasks. (Regardless of how many breaks are taken during the day, a 20-second microbreak can do wonders for increasing productivity.)

What you do during your microbreak depends on the position you're in for the majority of the day, but in most cases, good use of the time is to reset your posture. If your job requires repetitive motions, stretching or moving through a counter-posture for a few minutes (or even seconds) will help readjust your body. A quick mental and physical reset can mean the difference between injury and costly mistakes.

4. Try not to take work home

It's easy to properly get into the habit of taking work home when we're busy or have tight deadlines, but this should be the exception rather than the rule. When we prioritize getting the downtime we need for a healthy work-life balance, we can afford to pay full attention to those waiting for us at home. Suppose you must take work home, set aside a specific time to complete it – the earlier, the better.

5. Take holiday leave

Taking a complete break from work is beneficial to both mental and physical health. Taking a vacation can help you reduce work-related stress, prevent anxiety and depression, and improve your work performance and productivity. Employees taking leave is also in the best interests of employers.

Getting away from it all has been proven to be healthy for the mind, even for a short period. Lives have become increasingly hectic these days, and people desperately need to escape the constant stresses and challenges.

When you're on vacation, you can focus on having fun with family and friends and leave your daily worries behind. It doesn't matter if you're dipping your toes in a pool, soaking up the sun on a beach, doing something active, or experiencing some culture; all these activities will give you a wonderful mental boost.

Scientists have discovered that the psychological benefits can last up to a month after you return home. And why shouldn't everyone have the opportunity to enjoy a vacation? We at The Family Holiday Association believe that holidays should not be limited to the privileged and wealthy; we believe that everyone should benefit from holidays' mental health benefits.

Here are just a few of the numerous mental health benefits of vacations.

They help reduce stress

A study conducted by Nuffield Health, the UK's largest healthcare charity, and tour operator Kuoni discovered that not going on vacation has significant consequences. They discovered that those who did not take a vacation had higher blood pressure, slept less well, and were more stressed.

It's not surprising that vacations help us de-stress because we do things that make us happy and distract our minds. In addition, travel gives us a much-needed break from our hectic lifestyles, which helps us feel less stressed.

Holidays can make us mentally sharper and more creative

If your mind is emotionally exhausted, you are unlikely to function optimally. Just as you need to take breaks from work regularly to stay productive, you also need long breaks where you can properly rest.

Going on vacation can provide you with renewed motivation and the strength to carry on with your life when you return. According to one study, three days after a vacation, people felt more rested, less anxious, and happier.

Travel helps you stay active, which helps your mental health

It's common knowledge that exercise can improve your mental health. A long walk in a peaceful setting can do wonders for your mood. When we travel, we frequently have the opportunity to be active and explore new places, and we must travel on foot. Regular vacations where you have the opportunity to do something active, such as an activity or walking vacation, will undoubtedly help improve your mental health and overall well-being.

Travel broadens your mind, literally

Travel has been linked to increased creativity, cultural awareness, and personal growth, according to studies. Your brain goes into overdrive when you travel to new places. There are new sounds, sights, and smells to become accustomed to. Your brain absorbs your new surroundings, and you have interactions that help you become more culturally aware.

Traveling can provide you with something to look forward to.

According to research, simply having something to look forward to can help improve your mood. So, as soon as you click the 'book' button on that vacation website, your mind begins to do mental somersaults. Of course, everyone enjoys having a vacation to look forward to.

Travel can help depression

Using six days away from home as a guide, researchers from Mount Sinai's Icahn School of Medicine, the University of California, and Harvard discovered that this amount of time alters DNA, boosts the immune system, and reduces proteins linked to cognitive decline and depression. As a result, travel can provide a temporary respite and help nurse you back to mental health if you're feeling down or going through a particularly difficult period in your life.

6. Set realistic deadlines and deliver on them

If you plan your day, you will be able to spend more time doing high-quality work while exerting less effort. Therefore, it is critical to follow a process if you want to achieve your goals more effectively.

7. Sometimes, it's OK to say "No."

It's not always easy to say no. We all like to please our coworkers and be perceived as a "can-do" person at work, but we also have the right to set work limits when demands exceed our ability to deliver. You should not be afraid to say no and explain why. When you give a genuine response, it does not imply that you are failing your team. On the contrary, the task is more likely to be completed differently, and you'll be in a better position to say yes the next time.

8. Have a technology switch-off

Many of us are required to work outside of our normal working hours on occasion. But we all need time away from work to relax and unwind. Therefore, nobody should be expected to send and receive work emails at all hours of the day or night. Employees and managers must collaborate to avoid creating a culture of constant email checking.

Here are some email usage tips:

- Consider whether you need to be reachable 24 hours a day, seven days a week.
- If at all possible, avoid adding your work emails to your mobile phone.
- Try to be strict with yourself about checking your emails – don't make it a habit outside of work.
- Set a good example by not allowing late-night emails to become a part of your workplace culture.

Ask yourself who is driving any expectation of after-hours emailing – your manager, or do you enjoy feeling in demand? If you cannot respond to all urgent or important emails during your workday, this may indicate that your workload is too heavy. You should talk to your boss about it.

9. Make use of the Employee Assistance Program

Many employers provide an Employee Assistance Program or a similar program to help employees deal with personal and work-related issues that can impact their job performance, health, mental and emotional well-being. If your workplace provides a service, you may find it beneficial to speak with someone about something, especially if you are struggling. EAPs provide free, confidential, short-term counseling, referrals, and follow-up services.

10. Investigate appropriate flexible working arrangements.

Work flexible work arrangements enable many employees to increase their overall well-being by permitting them to find an arrangement that better fits their daily routine. Some laws help employees who meet certain criteria. These working arrangements must be negotiated with your employer. You must do your job efficiently and effectively that is acceptable to both you and your employer.

Flexible working arrangements can include the following:

- Working from home or in a more convenient location, rather than the office or worksite, allows greater flexibility.
- Flexible hours – beginning and ending times that can be changed to accommodate personal or family obligations
- Working longer days to make up for a shorter workweek is an example of a flexible pattern.
- Split shifts are possible with flexible rostering.
- Collaboration on the job
- Graduated return to work entails an employee returning to work part-time and gradually increasing

to full-time by an agreed-upon date (after parental leave or extended sick leave)
- Purchasing additional leave – for example, only 44 weeks of work in a year with the reduced salary payments spread across 52 weeks.

Our lifestyle

Eating healthily, getting enough sleep, exercising regularly, and avoiding harmful levels of alcohol and other drugs can help you maintain your mental health, manage anxiety and depression symptoms, and improve your overall well-being.

Exercise

Everyone knows that physical activity is critical for good health and well-being, but it can end up forgotten and neglected even with the best intentions. Stress management techniques, such as exercise, have been proven to be effective at treating mild to moderate depression and being a dependable way of handling stress.

There are numerous ways to become more active, including working out alone, with others, with a trainer, in classes, or with sports teams.

Relaxation

It is critical to make time for yourself to do something you enjoy. Connecting with the outside world and the pressures or demands on you might be as simple as clearing your electronic devices away, or it could be as difficult as spending time with your family or friends. A variety of relaxation techniques exist. Consider the positives in your life, especially those that help you unwind. It may be useful to keep a list of what works to refer to when needed.

Creative Ideas for Maintaining and Improving Well-Being keep physically fit

Take a walk or ride your bike

Cycling, for example, can lower your body's stress hormone, cortisol. Getting on your bike can also help to relieve tension in your body. According to research, those who cycle regularly have a significantly lower risk of feeling stressed.

Cycling can also be much less expensive in the long run than a gym membership, saving you money and relieving financial stress. Cycling and walking both stimulate the release of endorphins or "feel-good" hormones. These hormones aid in the relaxation of the mind and the enhancement of happiness. This improves your mood and reduces your anxiety.

Go swimming

Being physically active benefits mental health by improving mood, increasing self-esteem, lowering the risk of depression, slowing dementia and cognitive decline, improving sleep, and reducing stress.

Swimming has significantly reduced anxiety and depression symptoms in 1.4 million adults in the United Kingdom. In addition, swimming has reduced visits to a medical professional for mental health problems for nearly half a million British adults with mental health problems.

Do yoga or tai chi

Numerous studies have confirmed yoga's numerous mental and physical benefits. It can help you increase your strength and flexibility, reduce stress, depression, and anxiety, and improve your overall health by incorporating it into your routine. Practicing yoga once or twice per week could have a significant impact on your health.

Go to the gym

Exercise regularly can have a profoundly positive impact on depression, anxiety, and ADHD. It also reduces stress, improves memory, improves sleep, and improves your overall mood. Anyone can benefit from exercising, whether they are fitness enthusiasts or not. Small amounts of exercise can properly make a huge difference, according to research. Even sedentary or physically unfit people can learn to use exercise as a powerful tool to smoothly deal with mental health issues, improve their energy and outlook, and get more out of life.

Get good quality sleep. Pamper yourself

While research into the links between mental health and sleep is ongoing, current evidence suggests a bidirectional relationship. For example, sleeping problems are often exacerbated by mental health issues. At the same time, inadequate sleep, including insomnia, can contribute to worsening mental health problems.

Have a bubble bath

Throughout history, bathing has been about more than just personal hygiene. In ancient times, cleanliness was seen as a symbol of power and beauty, and baths were taken publicly to socialize and build communities.

Participants in a German study who soaked in a 40°C bath for 30 minutes reported an improvement in their mood. In fact, in this study, regular baths were more effective than aerobic exercise in treating depression.

Buy some flowers

You will feel less agitated after purchasing flowers from the market or placing them in your favorite vase—without even realizing it. Studies have shown flowers to stimulate creative energy and positive vibes, ultimately making us feel better.

Nature can change our moods and relieve stress. Flowers can help us overcome anxiety, depression, and the stresses of everyday life.

Lie on a beach

According to studies, spending time near the ocean is beneficial to one's health. For example, according to an analysis of English census data published in the journal Health Place, those who live near the coast have better physical and mental health than those who do not.

Get a massage

Massage can boost the production of endorphins like serotonin and dopamine. Endorphins are hormones that are released during times of happiness and relaxation. Due to the stress associated with a mental health problem, people with low endorphin levels are common. Endorphin deficiency has been linked to negative thoughts, anxiety, stress, and depression. Massage can increase the release of endorphins by stimulating the autonomic nervous system. An increase in endorphin levels, such as serotonin and dopamine, can make a person feel more positive, enthusiastic, and relaxed.

Read a book or magazine

Reading, according to a growing body of research, changes your mind.

MRI scans confirmed to Trusted Source that reading involves a complex network of circuits and signals in the brain. As your reading ability develops, these networks become stronger and more sophisticated.

Researchers used functional MRI scans to measure the effect of reading a novel on the brain in one study, Trusted Source, conducted in 2013. Over nine days, study participants read the novel "Pompeii." As the story progressed, more and more areas of the brain became active.

Brain scans revealed that brain connectivity increased throughout the reading period and for several days afterward, particularly in the somatosensory cortex, the part of the brain that responds to physical sensations such as movement and pain.

Write a letter or email

Going through cancer treatment can elicit a wide range of emotions, particularly concerning your relationships. Writing a letter to a loved one, whether you send it or not, can be a healthy way to properly express your feelings and say what's on your mind.

Letter writing differs from reflective or expressive writing in that you intend to express how you feel about your relationship or interactions with others.

Play a solo card game

Solitaire is a classic game that is known to relax your mind while also relaxing your body. While playing solitaire, you can enter a meditative state where you are relaxed and solely focused on the game. Solitaire can be useful for people who suffer from anxiety or have difficulty focusing because it properly keeps you focused and relaxed at the same time.

Do a crossword or sudoku

Sudoku, crossword puzzles, taking classes, reading, and writing are all brain games that can help delay dementia and Alzheimer's disease and protect the brain from decline. When you stretch your brain and try something new, especially when you use different parts of your brain and think differently, you're helping to sharpen and maintain your mind's sharpness.

Go to the movies or a market

Watching movies allows for emotional release. Even those who have difficulty expressing their emotions may find themselves laughing or crying during a movie. This emotional release can have a cathartic effect and make it easier for a person to express their emotions.

Pay a visit to a museum, art gallery, or library. In and around the house

The advantages of museums extend far beyond simply imparting knowledge. While learning is important from a purely practical and academic standpoint, there is a significant psychological component that we must never overlook. For those who seek refuge and solace in creative environments, we should value museums' ability to reduce feelings of anxiety, isolation, and depression in their visitors. Furthermore, we see an increasing number of examples of museums actively working to improve mental health in local communities, with excellent results.

Cook something new

According to one study, a little creativity and creation in the kitchen can make people happier. According to the findings of the study, published in the Journal of Positive Psychology, people who regularly engage in small, creative projects like baking or cooking report feeling more relaxed and happier in their daily lives.

Listen to music or the radio

Music can change the brain. Music, according to neuroscientists, causes the release of several neurochemicals that play a role in brain function and mental health: dopamine, a chemical associated with pleasure and "reward" centers, stress hormones such as cortisol, serotonin, and other hormones related to immunity.

oxytocin, a neurotransmitter that promotes the ability to connect with others

Although more research is properly needed to understand how music can be used therapeutically to treat mental illness, some studies Trusted Source suggest that music therapy can improve people with schizophrenia's quality of life and social connectedness.

Play in the backyard with your children

She claims that play can "promote positive feelings like joy and excitement, which can bolster mood and diminish anxiety and sadness." But, in the meantime, insufficient playtime has been shown to increase symptoms of depression, anxiety, inattention, and behavioral problems in students, she claims.

Do some gardening

There is mounting evidence that gardening can improve our mental health, which is important when the NHS is overburdened. A mental illness affects one out of every four adults.

According to research conducted in Sweden*, the more people who used their gardens, the less stress they experienced.

According to a study published in the Mental Health Journal*, gardening can reduce stress, improve mood, and reduce symptoms of depression and anxiety.

Practical strategies for improving sleep:

- Caffeine, nicotine, and alcohol should be reduced or eliminated.
- Maintain a consistent sleep schedule – even on weekends.
- Avoid naps, which can disrupt your sleep quality.
- Exercise, preferably first thing in the morning. Ascertain that you have a comfortable sleeping environment. Make sure your bedroom isn't too hot—cool temperatures help you fall and stay asleep.
- There will be no phones, televisions, or laptop computers in the bedroom.
- Try to relax and slow down for at least 30 minutes before going to bed.
- Look for ways to properly lessen the negative impact of shiftwork on your sleep quality and quantity.

Our social relationships

Good mental health is supported by healthy relationships, whereas social isolation and poor relationships can be risk factors for mental health conditions such as anxiety and depression. Good, open, and regular communication is an important part of developing strong relationships. This can be accomplished by discussing your thoughts and feelings with family, friends, and trusted coworkers. Some people find it natural and easy to share personal information. Others may require the assistance of a health professional or a community group to feel more comfortable opening up.

The size of your social network is less important than the quality of your relationships. Having a supportive network with whom you can relax, have fun, and lean on when tough times are linked to good mental health.

Ways to stay connected

If we suffer from a mental illness, our instinct may be to withdraw and avoid our friends. On the other hand, friendships can play an important role in helping us live with or recover from a mental health problem, as well as overcome the isolation that often comes with it. We can form the strongest bonds with those who have helped us through difficult times.

Friendship is an important factor in maintaining our mental health. Our friends can help us stay grounded, put things into perspective, and deal with the problems that life throws at us.

If you don't know who to call, reach out to acquaintances and neighbors

Because we are social creatures, social connection is essential to our health and overall well-being. In addition, being together has some immediate advantages: People who are part of a connected community eat healthier, are less likely to smoke, are more likely to participate in physical activities, and are more likely to engage in overall healthy behaviors.

On the other hand, loneliness has significant health consequences that are comparable to the effects of diabetes and heart disease on the cardiovascular system.

Don't be afraid to greet strangers with a smile and a hello

The growing body of literature indicates that engaging with and trusting strangers benefits our well-being, the well-being of those we meet, and the health of society. For example, in the United States, friendly behavior toward strangers has been linked to higher self-esteem in teenagers. Greater trust in strangers has been linked to improved overall health in China. Furthermore, trust in strangers has been linked to individual happiness in Canada.

Reduce your time spent in front of the television or computer

Many people use their screens until they fall asleep, scrolling through social media, reading articles, or watching their favorite show. According to research, increased screen time is associated with decreased sleep quality and sleep duration. This is especially noticeable in children and adolescents who have screens (TVs, computers, tablets) in their bedrooms and have access to them before going to sleep. Inadequate sleep, either in terms of quality or duration, has been linked to worsening various mental health conditions, including anxiety. Turning off (or limiting the use of) electronic devices at least 15-30 minutes before going to bed can help prevent any negative effects of technology and screen use on sleep.

Join regular networking, social, or special interest community groups.

To thrive in life, we need the company of others, and the strength of our bonds has a significant impact on our mental health and happiness. Being socially connected to others can alleviate stress, anxiety, and depression, boost self-esteem, bring comfort and prevent loneliness, joy, and even add years to your life.

Consider volunteering, which allows you to help others while also allowing you to meet new people

Volunteering has been shown in studies to reduce depression rates, particularly among people aged 65 and up. Furthermore, volunteering promotes social interaction and forming a support network based on common interests, both of which have been properly shown to reduce depression.

Bring your kids or pets to the park or playground

Spend much more time in parks and green spaces can help
with the treatment of mental health issues like depression,
anxiety, and stress. Ensuring that everyone has access to
parks and outdoor programming is a critical way to increase
your community's positive effects on health and quality of
life.

Our thoughts

Many studies show that psychological therapies can help us manage how we think and behave. These therapies recognize that by changing our thinking and approach problems rationally, we can shift from pessimistic or unhelpful thoughts and reactions to more beneficial problem-solving approaches.

Learning the connection between thoughts and feelings

Situation

Consider a recent experience that was upsetting or difficult for you. For example, after I asked him to change something in a document, my colleague was abrupt and dismissive.

Mood

What were your emotions like? How intense was this state of mind? (From 0% to 100%) E.g., 80% of the people were hurt. 90% of the people are enraged. Eighty percent of the time, I'm frustrated. Thinking that is counterproductive

What were your thoughts like? When we talk to ourselves the way we do, it's unhelpful and contributes to feelings of failure.

Thinking in terms of black and white – "I have to finish everything before I go home, or everything will be a disaster."

What-ifs? – "What if I put in all this effort and still fail?" Then, I'll never be able to look someone in the eyes again."

Spiral of negatives –"Thus, I am useless." I have bad news to report."

Jumping to conclusions – "My colleague was very direct with me. He must be irritated by what I said at the meeting."

Oversimplification – "That client has threatened to take his business elsewhere." All of my clients must be dissatisfied."

Looking too far ahead – "Negative consequences are likely to result if this doesn't go well."

Strong, unwavering words – "I should..., I must..., I always..., I never......"

Unkind or cruel to oneself – "I'm a failure, I'm stupid, I'm a fraud... someone will see through me one day and realize I'm not all that great after all."

Unhelpful thoughts must be challenged.

Ask yourself the following questions:

- What would I say if a close friend or someone I cared about was thinking this way?
- Will I see things differently in five years when I look back?
- Is the information I'm basing my conclusions on backed up by evidence?

- What are the weaknesses I am ignoring, and how am I handling them?

Helpful thinking

Write alternative, more balanced thoughts that could have been more beneficial. E.g., He isn't always like this. Maybe he's stressed out because of his divorce, and it has nothing to do with me. Perhaps I should just ask how he's doing.

New mood

After you've practiced helpful thoughts, rate your moods again. Make a list of any new moods (0-100 percent), E.g., 10% of the people are hurt. 10% are enraged. 20% are dissatisfied.

Symptoms of common mental health conditions

Anxiety

Anxiety symptoms frequently emerge gradually over time. Because we all have some anxiety, it can be difficult to know how much is too much. Anxiety disorders must have a significant impact on a person's life to be diagnosed. There are various types of anxiety, each with its own set of symptoms. Anxiety symptoms include hot and cold flushes, a racing heart, chest tightening, excessive fear or worry, obsessive thinking, and compulsive behavior.

Depression

While we all feel sad, depressed, or discouraged from time to time, these feelings don't pass for some people. Instead, they may persist, weeks, months, or even years later, regardless of any apparent cause.

Conclusion

Physical and mental health should be taken care of while in college, so learning how to take care of both is as important as learning how to take care of the other. This relationship is well known: mentally healthy people are healthier physically. To determine whether someone is mentally healthy, you must determine whether they recognize their abilities, can cope with the stresses of daily life properly, and contribute to their community.

Mental health is not necessarily linked to happiness or success. Even the most healthful individuals will experience bouts of depression, loneliness, or anxiety from time to time. However, they can manage these feelings, overcome them, and move on. Although mild feelings or moods are usually nothing to worry about, when they persist and interfere with normal functioning, it could be a sign of a more serious mental health problem and prompt an evaluation to see if professional help is needed.

A mental disorder or medical condition marked by significant "changes in thinking, mood, or behavior (or some combination thereof) associated with stress and associated difficulties in functioning" is referred to as "mental illness." depression is the most common mental illness in the United States, affecting nearly one-quarter of the adult population. According to forecasts, depression will rank second behind only ischemic heart disease as a cause of disability by 2020.

Indications indicate that psychological disorders, such as depression, are frequently coupled with other diseases and risk behaviors, including type 2 diabetes, various cancers, cardiovascular disease, asthma, and a myriad of unhealthy lifestyle habits, such as inactivity, smoking, and excessive drinking. That is to say, if you are mentally unhealthy, you are more likely to suffer from disease and ill health. Because of this, it is equally important to take care of your mental health while you are in college as it is to take care of your physical health. There is a strong connection between the two: good mental health contributes to overall health. The main focus of mental health is maintaining the ability to do things in the context of life's normal stresses.

You do not have to be happy or successful to have good mental health. Mental illness is not reserved for a small number of people. For the majority of people, it presents as feelings of depression, loneliness, or anxiety. These are all feelings that people in good mental health can contend with and overcome. A chronic, long-term emotional state can sometimes indicate the need for help.

When people have a mental illness, it is common for their emotions, feelings, and thoughts to become unpredictable or severely out of control. More than 26% of the adult population in the United States has depression. Depression is expected to be the second most disabling condition worldwide by 2020, with ischemic heart disease remaining the leading cause.

Studies indicate that both depression and a wide range of chronic diseases, including diabetes, cancer, cardiovascular disease, asthma, and obesity, are closely tied to the development and progression of many chronic diseases, as well as a wide range of chronic disease risk behaviors, such as inactivity, smoking, excessive drinking, and insufficient sleep. In another way, those with poor mental and physical health may be more vulnerable to disease. So, since learning how to take care of your mental health while in college is just as important as learning how to take care of your physical health, you should understand how to do both of these things.

Being happy or successful does not necessarily mean that you have good mental health. Most people have had times when they've felt depressed, lonely, or anxious, but mentally healthy people can handle these feelings and get over them. Such feelings or moods might continue for a while, but when they get in the way of someone's normal functioning, it is a sign of a more serious mental health problem.

"Mental illness" is defined as the "affecting of the mind, mood, or behavior with some level of dysfunction and also may be accompanied by additional signs and symptoms, such as changes in thinking, mood, or behavior (or some combination thereof)." Mental illness affects over 26% of adults in the United States. The second-leading cause of disability in the world, after ischemic heart disease, is predicted to be depression by 2020.

Research indicates that a wide range of diseases, such as diabetes, cancer, cardiovascular disease, asthma, and obesity, as well as a variety of disease risk behaviors, such as inactivity, smoking, excessive drinking, and insufficient sleep, are connected to mental disorders, particularly depression. Alternatively, if you are mentally unhealthy, you are more likely to contract a disease and be physically unhealthy.

Visit And Buy the Other Books of This Author

Happy Saint Patrick's Day: Saint Patrick's Day Planner/Journal with 8.5x11 inches and 100 Pages

https://www.amazon.com/dp/B09BY841SZ

St. Patrick's Day: Saint Patrick's Day Planner/Journal with 8.5x11 inches and 100 Pages

https://www.amazon.com/dp/B09BY7XWGD

Happy Easter: Easter Egg Patterns Worksheet: 8.5x11 Inches 60 Pages

https://www.amazon.com/dp/B09BT2B6F3

Easter Hunt Activity Happy Easter: Easter Hunt Activity Journal | Notebook size 8.5x11 60 Pages

https://www.amazon.com/dp/B09BY7XWKL

Easter Day Spring Writing Assignment worksheet: Easter Day Spring Writing Assignment worksheet | 8.5x11 60 Pages | Spring Worksheet

https://www.amazon.com/dp/B09BY5HNVB

Cinco De Mayo: Large Updated Organizer with Daily Spreads For 2 Months with Cover Paperback https://www.amazon.com/dp/B09BY8178L

Taking full charge of your finance: Easy Guide to Personal Finance

https://www.amazon.com/Taking-full-charge-your-finance/dp/B099C8S85Z

Sure, Steps to Wealth Creation: How to Build Wealth from Nothing

https://www.amazon.com/Sure-Steps-Wealth-Creation-Nothing/dp/B099C3GNQH

All You Need to Know About Cryptocurrency: Understanding Risk and Reward in Investing

https://www.amazon.com/Need-Know-About-Cryptocurrency-Understanding/dp/B099C3GNML

Eliminating Your Debt in 12 (x) Easy Steps and Keep Them Off: A Practical Guide to Eliminating Your Debt Forever!

https://www.amazon.com/Eliminating-Your-Debt-Easy-Steps/dp/B099BZX4FX

NLP For Beginners

https://www.amazon.com/NLP-Beginners-RS-Johnson-ebook/dp/B098JBH28Q

Credit Repair Secrets

44

<-*END*->